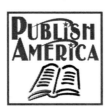

PublishAmerica
Baltimore

GU00707285

First printing

PublishAmerica has allowed this work to remain exactly as the author intended, verbatim, without editorial input.

Softcover 978-1-4489-6869-5
PAperback 978-1-4512-4802-9
PUBLISHED BY PUBLISHAMERICA, LLLP
www.publishamerica.com
Baltimore

Printed in the United States of America

Dedication

For Jon
My friend, my partner,
and the love of my life

Acknowledgements

Human beings, who are almost unique in having the ability to learn from the experience of others, are also remarkable for their apparent disinclination to do so. ~Douglas Adams

I have traveled many roads in my life, with many destinations, some good, some not so good. Along the way, I've met a lot of people, and learned a lot of lessons. People rarely learn from the mistakes of others—we generally insist, knowingly or otherwise, on making our own. I don't seek to keep you from your lessons, nor from the personal growth they can bring, but perhaps this book can help to shorten the learning curve that comes after.

As was always said at the end of my Al-Anon meetings, "take what you need and leave the rest." As with treatments, not everything will work for everyone. However, there are some Fibromyalgia-related experiences that are common to most of us, and there are some solutions that will work for many of us.

Thanks are due to my husband and biggest cheerleader, Jon, for support, encouragement, and the occasional editing and suggestions for improvement. This is a much better book because he gave it a reality check. There are so many people I should thank, but in fear of leaving someone out, I won't list them all here. You know who you are, and you know I couldn't have done this without you. Special thanks to my dear friend Laurel Hughlett for her calm, no-nonsense style of friendship and support, which keeps me sane and grounded when I'm in danger of bouncing off the walls.

I also want to thank the members of the Daily Strength Fibromyalgia Community (www.dailystrength.org), as well as the members of the Richmond Fibromyalgia Support Group, for sharing their thoughts, their feelings, and their own solutions for coping day-to-day. These generous souls have been an invaluable resource in writing this book, and in the process of getting to know them and learning from them, I am proud to say that a number of them have become my friends. We have shared the joy of births, the sorrow of deaths, and the small triumphs and failures of everyday life that make up our existence. Without their support and their willingness to share their lives with me, this book might never have been. There are too many to mention individually—but if you're in one of those groups, know that I appreciate you more than mere words can say.

This is not a scholarly dissertation. It's just a little book of words I would say to you if we were sitting at my dining room table having coffee. I have tried to keep the writing conversational, in the hope that you, the reader, will have a sense of talking with a friend, rather than sitting through a lecture.

My further hope is that, in reading this book, you will find at least one suggestion that you can apply to your own situation. If one idea or concept from this book makes your living with Fibromyalgia a little bit easier, than I have fulfilled my goal in writing it.

Taming the
Fibromyalgia Dragon

Thoughts on Life with Fibromyalgia

Friends

"What do we live for, if it is not to make life less difficult for each other?" ~George Eliot

Friends—first, and most important, to have one, you must be one. In order to make and nurture lasting friendships, you must be someone who others will want to be friends with. That doesn't mean you must be able to participate in any or all of the activities your friends enjoy. Friendship is not dependent on activity—it's only dependent on keeping in touch. It's not necessary to a friendship that you always be able to physically participate. It *is* necessary to accept that all modern communication devices work two ways.

You don't have to wait for your friends to contact you—everybody is busy—if you want to talk, then call, or email, or even text your friends, and ask what's up with them. Thanks to these modern methods of keeping in touch, there is no longer any excuse for not checking in with the people you care about, no matter how much fibro is kicking your butt on any given day.

When you talk with your friends, keep the conversation centered on ideas, interests, and activities—the common ground that brought you together to begin with. Spare them the details of your latest test results, or your latest mysterious symptom. Find a support group for that. With your friends, talk about the things you have always talked about, whether it's school, careers, family, politics, it doesn't matter what the topic is, as long as it's not about you and your Fibromyalgia. It's not that they don't care—if they're really your friends they *do* care, but that doesn't mean they want to hear every detail.

Plan conversational topics ahead of time to avoid falling into the trap of discussing your health for hours on end. When you're spending time with a friend, consider ahead of time what shared interests or common ground you can talk about. Example: If you, or they, have just had a baby, you might talk about how fast kids grow, and how you just found the cutest little shoes you've ever seen.

In terms of what *not* to talk about, think of it this way— when you're discussing babies, you don't share the lurid details of the contents of the diaper you just changed.

Family*

When our relatives are at home, we have to think of all their good points or it would be impossible to endure them. ~George Bernard Shaw

A lot of family relationships can be maintained in the same manner as friendships (see "Friends"). However, there are some differences. Family members often have a sense of "entitlement" to your personal information. It's important to remember that their feeling of entitlement does not obligate you to satisfy their curiosity.

It's not only OK, it's often desirable to keep the details of your condition to yourself. If you have a supportive family, you can measure how much Fibromyalgia-related information they can assimilate by their reaction to anything you choose to share. Watch their faces. If their eyes are glazing over, or they're squirming, eyes wandering as if they are seeking an escape, change the subject—preferably to what's going on in *their* life.

On the other hand, if they seem *too* interested in the details of your health, to the point where you feel it's invasive, you might invoke your own version of a tried and true "Dear Abby" line, "Now why on earth would you want to know *that?*"

There is a fine line between enough information and too much. How much is too much is going to vary, depending on personalities and relationships. In the end, only you can make that decision, but in making it, you might consider the following:

- Did they ask about your health? (It doesn't count if they only said "How are you?")
- If you started talking about your health, did they seem interested? (or did they look trapped?)

If the answer to either of those questions is "No," you may have crossed that fine, invisible line into the land of "Too Much Information."

Does not apply to a spouse or life partner—that will take a whole book to address.

Well-Meant Comments

If you judge people, you have no time to love them. ~Mother Teresa

I choose to believe that most people are kind, caring, and compassionate. With that belief comes the assumption that, when people make comments about my health, they mean well. The following are some of the well-meant comments I have either heard, or had related to me by others with Fibromyalgia:

- Everyone has pain somewhere…
- Fibromyalgia is just what doctors say when they don't know what you really have.
- I had that, and I was cured by…
- Pain meds don't help people with Fibromyalgia.
- Oh, I read about that! It's caused by…
- There's a pill for that now!
- You just have to push through the pain!

Each of these comments, and others like them, has the ability to create stress for the Fibromyalgia patient to whom it is said. We can't choose all of the people in our lives, and we can't always succeed in convincing the people in our lives that what we feel is not what they feel, or what they've experienced.

I truly believe that when *most* people make *most* of these comments, they are trying to relate to us by relating our condition to something they understand. While the comments may be poorly chosen, and the information they are relying on inaccurate, if you tell yourself that they mean well, it's often easier to deflect the comments and avoid the stress of trying to change what they believe.

It's pointless to argue with people who hold these viewpoints. No matter how tempting it is to try to convince them of the errors in their thinking, it is a waste of your precious time and limited energy. It may also serve to damage a relationship that you want to preserve.

Let it go—move on—don't give them power by letting their comments get under your skin. Seriously—let it go.

Treatments and Medication

"If anybody said that I should die if I did not take beef-tea or mutton, even under medical advice, I would prefer death" ~Mahatma Gandhi

While there is, for now, no cure for Fibromyalgia, there are many treatment options for the symptoms. Each individual has a preferred approach to treatment. Many choose to seek an "all natural" path, while others turn to conventional medicine for solutions.

How you approach the management of your symptoms is a very personal issue for which you should not be criticized or judged. Remember, when you discuss treatment options with others who have Fibromyalgia, that they have exactly the same right as you to make their own health care decisions. It's never OK to judge someone for the treatment choices they make—never.

When others who do not have Fibromyalgia ask about your treatment, suspect that they are seeking conversational fodder rather than inquiring about your well-being. You will make your own choice about how much to share, but keep these points in mind. They may come in handy if someone feels the need to comment on your treatment choices:

- All medications have side effects, and some are more troublesome than others. If you choose prescription or over-the-counter medication as your treatment of choice, educate yourself about the side effects of the medication you (or your doctor) choose. Doctors know the most common side effects. You need to know all of them.
- The fact that a medication is sold over the counter does not mean it's either safe for long-term use or without side effects.
- Don't assume that a substance is safe just because it's "natural." By way of example, I submit, for your consideration, poison ivy and hemlock. In addition, many "natural" substances have their own side effects, and/or can interact with other medications, herbs, and supplements. Always be sure to educate yourself on both side effects and interactions. They are all chemicals— whether manufactured or naturally occurring.
- There is very little chance of becoming addicted to any drug if you do not have a history of substance abuse.

Addiction is the compulsive use of a substance to treat emotional/spiritual pain. Using pain medication of any kind to treat chronic physical pain, whether you take one pill or many more each day, does not constitute addiction.

•   Physical dependence is not addiction. Many of the common medications useful for treating pain, and some sleep aids, have the potential to create a physical dependence in your body. All that means is that, if you or your doctor decide you need to discontinue a medication on which you have become physically dependent, you must wean off of that drug gradually, rather than stopping "cold turkey," in order to diminish or avoid withdrawal symptoms. That's really all it means.

•   Some alternative treatments that have proved helpful to many with Fibromyalgia include:

> •   Acupuncture
> •   Herbal and/or Vitamin/Mineral Supplements
> •   Massage
> •   Water Aerobics or other pool exercise
> •   Yoga—there are modified poses that work well for the physically challenged
> •   Medical marijuana (where legal)

- Some things you may want to avoid, unless your doctor specifically recommends them:
  - "Detox" products
  - Overly complex regimens for which you can't verify peer-reviewed research showing benefits, especially if they are very expensive
  - Any organization or practitioner claiming to have a "cure" for Fibromyalgia. When there is a real cure, nobody will be keeping it a secret.

Buyer beware—the world is full of unscrupulous people who take advantage of the desperation of people in pain. If it seems too good to be true, it probably is.

Abuse

"Domestic violence causes far more pain than the visible marks of bruises and scars. It is devastating to be abused by someone that you love and think loves you in return" ~Dianne Feinstein

Let me say first that I have very strong feelings about this topic. I have lived in an abusive relationship, and no one should have to live that way. I don't care who you are, who you're with, or what you've done. Nothing you can ever do will justify being physically, emotionally, or sexually abused.

The following are "warning signs" that your relationship may be heading in a dangerous direction*:

- Extreme jealousy
- Constant put-downs
- Telling you what you can and can't do
- Possessiveness or controlling behavior

- Financial control
- Making false accusations
- Keeping you from seeing or talking with friends and family

Not all of the above signs will be in every relationship. These are some other things to consider that, taken in combination with the above warning signs, may indicate that your relationship is heading in an unhealthy, or even dangerous direction*:

- History of abusive behavior, especially against a former dating or marital partner
- Big mood swings
- Explosive temper
- Belief that abuse is acceptable in relationships

Now that we've got some definitions in place, let's talk about what this has to do with Fibromyalgia. The reason I included this information is pretty simple. People who have a chronic medical condition often have self-esteem issues related to their inability, or perceived inability, to live like "normal people." They are often easy to manipulate, and when a controlling individual says "Who else would put up with you?" or "Who would love you if I leave?" they honestly believe the answer is "nobody."

I don't know you—but there are things I do know. First, no one has the right to abuse any other person. Second, it is never, ever OK to take advantage of anyone, physically, financially, emotionally, or sexually. Last, but certainly not least, love doesn't hurt. Love feels warm, and fun, and safe. If you are being abused, it's not love. It doesn't matter what you've done, or how sick you may be. If you're being hurt, it's not love.

*Adapted from www.thesafeplace.org

Resources for Domestic Abuse Information and Assistance:

http://www.ndvh.org/

http://www.thesafeplace.org/

National Domestic Violence Hotline (Anonymous & Confidential Help 24/7)

1.800.799.SAFE (7233) 1.800.787.3224 (TTY)

http://www.da.usda.gov/shmd/aware.htm

For those outside the U.S., google "Domestic Violence <your country>" (without quotes or brackets)

Choices

"In the long run, we shape our lives, and we shape ourselves. The process never ends until we die. And the choices we make are ultimately our responsibility." ~Eleanor Roosevelt

This is a topic that, while seemingly innocuous, often creates dissension. I'm going to ask you to just go with me for now, and you can make your own decisions (as always) later.

You have choices. Everyone has choices. The fact that you may not *like* the choices that are available to you at any given time doesn't mean you don't have them. If you are a person of legal age, wherever you are, then you do have choices.

So…why is that important, you might ask? This book is about living with Fibromyalgia—I didn't choose to have it— so why is this so important? The answer is really simple, but this is where the dissension comes in. The thing I need you to accept is that, wherever you are right now, you choose to be there. Before you get up and throw this book in the trash, again, just go with me for a few minutes. Give the thought some time to sit quietly.

I am *not*—absolutely positively *not*—saying you chose to have Fibromyalgia, or any other health issues. What I am saying is that we have choices in most areas of our life. Health is an exception—and to a degree we even have choices there, as some health conditions are tied to lifestyle choices. But I digress.

The thought I'm trying to get you to think is that you choose to be where you are, and you choose to be with whoever you're with. The reason it's important to accept this is that, as soon as you do, you are no longer a victim. When you accept that you are with a person, or in a place, or doing whatever work you do, because of choices you've made, it allows you to see the whole world through different eyes.

I could go on with this topic for hours, but because others have done it so much better, I'm going to recommend that you read *How To Be Your Own Best Friend*, by Bernard Berkowitz and Mildred Newman. This small, quick read changed my life—it might change yours as well.

Changes

If you don't like something change it; if you can't change it, change the way you think about it. ~Mary Engelbreit

There is a wonderful little story by Emily Perl Kingsley called *"Welcome to Holland,"* written for parents of children with disabilities, The premise of the story is this: If you spend all of your time mourning because things didn't turn out the way you expected, you will miss the beauty of your new circumstances. *"Different"* is not automatically defined as bad or good; different is often just different. You may be unable to do some, even many, of the things you used to do. That doesn't mean there is *nothing* you can do.

Think about the things you really enjoyed doing before Fibromyalgia became a factor. Were they physical? If so, what changes can you make to the way you do them, to allow you to continue, or to start over, and do those things differently? Or—find another physical pursuit you *can* do.

Example: Maybe you loved to run each day after work, but now you can't run for as long, or as far, as before, or maybe you're too tired or in too much pain to run at all. Change that run to a relaxing walk. You'll enjoy the scenery more, and your body will thank you for the exercise. By changing your perspective, it's possible that you can continue to do many of the things you used to enjoy by adapting them to accommodate your pain and energy levels.

If the things you enjoyed were creative, intellectual, or both, you may find that those things also need to be done differently. "Fibro fog" is a very real attribute of Fibromyalgia. Your attention span may be diminished, and it may take longer to process information. For some, short-term memory is affected. These are very real challenges, but they can be overcome with some adjustments in how you do things.

If your attention span is shorter than it used to be, break tasks down into smaller "bites" and take regular breaks. This may also help if you are having trouble processing information. Don't struggle and force yourself to "stay on task." While that may be good advice for others, it doesn't usually work well when dealing with a cognitive deficit. Forcing yourself to keep pushing on will lead to frustration, and frustration can take all the fun out of a pastime you used to enjoy.

Short term memory, while a significant challenge, may be the easiest of the "fog" related issues to overcome. Keep a pen and a small pad (or PDA) with you at all times. When you set an appointment, make plans to meet a friend, or decide what to fix for dinner, write it down. Once you have made the note to yourself, you can go on to other things without fear of forgetting something important.

Take a look around—the sun is still shining, children are still laughing, and if you listen closely, you will hear the sounds of nature around you—unless, like me, you live near an Interstate highway, in which case the sounds you hear will be horns and engines. But again I digress.

My point is, the whole world has not changed because of your diagnosis. The things that were beautiful before are still beautiful. The sights and sounds that you enjoyed before have not changed. Turn on the music, listen to the birds, or the laughter of children. Tune in to the color, sound, and scents of a sunny spring morning.

It may not be the "destination" you set out to find, but if you only focus on what you've lost, you'll miss out on what you still have. It's different for each person—the equation of loss and what remains—so it's up to you to figure out what that means in your individual case.

Find the beauty, comfort, and value in what you have—don't look back—look forward.

Exercise

There's no easy way out. If there were, I would have bought it. And believe me, it would be one of my favorite things! ~Oprah Winfrey

If you're still reading—I'm going to assume you at least have an open mind on this topic. I'm not going to belabor the point, as I understand that telling someone who is in pain to do something that, in their perception, will cause more pain— well let's just say the person doing the telling isn't going to win any popularity contests.

However, the data is clear, and the facts, no matter how little we like them, are indisputable. People with Fibromyalgia function better, and even feel better, when they get some exercise on a regular basis. This doesn't mean you have to run out, join a gym, and try to look like your next-door neighbor who never had an ounce of fat on her body to begin with. It just means you will feel better if you move around enough to keep your muscles toned. There are many ways to accomplish this, and the challenge is to find an activity that 1) you find reasonably enjoyable, and 2) doesn't cause you to have a symptom "flare."

One form of exercise you might consider is water aerobics. The support and buoyancy of the water cushions the entire body so that any exercise is extremely low-impact, and if the water is warm, so much the better. This is a form of exercise recommended by many doctors for their patients with Fibromyalgia, and I have heard good things from people who are actually doing it. Those who have tried it, and stuck with it, swear by it, and they tell me they have more pain if they don't exercise regularly for some reason, such as illness or schedule conflicts. If you aren't ready for organized aerobics (and I confess that I'm not), consider going to a pool and just walking in the water. The water will provide both a cushion and some resistance to your movements, at the same time softening the impact and giving you a better workout.

Another benefit of keeping muscles toned is that you are not so likely to hurt yourself doing routine daily tasks. If the muscles are not toned, it is much easier to injure yourself doing "normal" activities, such as lifting a small child or taking out the trash.

As I said earlier, I won't belabor the point—take it or leave it—but I strongly recommend trying to find something you enjoy enough to stick with it for a bit, to see if it helps you.

Work

Disability is a matter of perception. If you can do just one thing well, you're needed by someone. ~Martina Navratilova

Working with Fibromyalgia can create a multitude of issues for both employee and employer. Some issues are related to changes in cognitive function; others may be related to pain, and/or the medication used to manage pain. The solutions to these issues, while they are not simple, are often possible if employer and employee work together to define, and then accommodate* these issues.

The specific accommodation(s) available are too many and varied to list here, but by way of suggestion, I'll mention several of the most common changes, most of which are reasonably priced (or even free) and within the reach of even the smallest employer's budget:

Breaks—By taking short breaks, a person with Fibromyalgia may be able to recharge their batteries, both mental and physical, making them more alert and productive.

Adaptive Technology—There are many small and inexpensive devices that can make working with Fibromyalgia much more comfortable. Those devices include, but are not limited to:

- wrist wrest for keyboard and/or mouse
- adjustable foot rest
- ergonomic keyboard
- lumbar support pillow
- voice recognition software
- telephone headset
- properly fitted adjustable chair**

Flexible schedules and telecommuting are two options to explore if the job is suitable for either. The nature of some types of work is that the worker must be on site, or at least in a particular place, at a particular time. The receptionist who answers phones and directs calls can do that job from anywhere with a little bit of creativity and modern technology. A teacher can, in some instances, teach from a remote location. However, the person who quality checks products coming off an assembly line, the police officer who patrols the streets, or the dentist who takes care of your teeth, must be in the right place, at the right time, in order to perform the task. An evaluation of a particular job will reveal whether telecommuting or flexible scheduling are reasonable accommodations.

Having said all of that, as an experienced HR professional, I urge you to do a reality check on your own situation before pursuing accommodation. The law is clear, but not all employers will be willing to work to find accommodations that will provide a better working situation for a disabled employee. If you don't feel that your employer will voluntarily participate in a discussion about disability accommodations, be careful of how (or whether) you approach the subject. The reality is that there are some employers who would rather risk legal action than cooperate with an employee's accommodation request.

If you feel that may be the case, consider consulting with an employment law attorney before making an accommodation request, so that you have a "Plan B" if you don't get a good response from your employer. Each situation is different— you are the only one who can make the call on what the risks and rewards of an accommodation request may be.

*The Americans With Disabilities Act may determine whether accommodation is mandated in each case. For advice specific to your situation, consult a human resources professional or an employment law attorney.

**The specific chair needed may be out of reach of a small company's budget.

Education

"Each handicap is like a hurdle in a steeplechase, and when you ride up to it, if you throw your heart over, the horse will go along, too."
~Lawrence Bixby

I include this topic because I firmly believe that education gives you options you would not otherwise have. The career I have, by virtue of having prepared myself through education, offers me a great deal of autonomy, flexibility, and even privacy by virtue of a private office, that I probably would not have otherwise. I directly credit these "perks" of management with my continued ability to work despite the challenges of Fibromyalgia.

A lot of the information on workplace accommodation also applies to the educational setting. Most large public universities, as well as community colleges, have a person or department dedicated to working with students with disabilities to enable them to pursue their educational goals. If such a person or department is not readily available, inquire in the Admissions office—they should be able to point you in the right direction.

If you are an adult considering returning to school, take a good look at all of your options. I completed my degree in 1998, and the entire educational landscape has changed since then. I was fortunate to be in the right place just as non-traditional "adult degree programs" were coming into the mainstream of higher education. I completed my first four semesters at a community college, one class at a time, over a period of more than ten years. With a non-traditional adult degree program offered by an accredited institution, I was able to complete my last two years in the normal two-year period, meeting once a week and doing most of the work on my own schedule, outside of the formal classroom setting.

The option of entirely on-line learning is now available, and the offerings are both plentiful and varied. If you choose to go this route (and it may be ideal for many with Fibromyalgia), carefully screen the schools you are considering. There are, and always will be, some "diploma mills" out there that will sell you a diploma without your doing the course work to earn it. That may be very tempting if you doubt your ability to stand up to the rigors of higher education, but don't—please don't do it.

These schools are known to employers and others. Their degrees are valueless, and all you'll have in the end is a very expensive piece of wall art.

Explore your options—non-traditional programs and on-line learning are available from well-known, accredited universities. Don't be misled by something that seems too easy. Good options are available, but know that, with or without accommodation, you will have to do the work in order to come away from the process with credentials of value.

Belief/Spirituality

"Faith is taking the first step even when you don't see the whole staircase." ~Dr. Martin Luther King Jr.

Spirituality is not the same as "religion" or even "faith." You can be a spiritual person without either. It is, however, an essential element of many people's psychological well-being. It seems to become more so when situations of health and/or mortality arise. Being diagnosed with an incurable condition, even when it's not life-threatening, causes many to ask questions and seek answers that they were not concerned with before the diagnosis. It may also cause one to question the answers they accepted before they were diagnosed with Fibromyalgia.

If you follow a specific faith tradition, and it provides you with hope and comfort, then you are probably on the right path *for you*. If you do not follow a specific faith tradition, and you either don't feel the need, or don't feel a strong calling to any particular set of beliefs, that may be the right path for you—at least for now. This isn't something you can force or fake—it has to come from inside—has to feel right and real—in order to provide a sense of comfort and meaning.

As we grow personally and learn more about the essential nature of the world around us, many people come to believe in a power greater than themselves, whether or not they give that power a name. The complexity of ecology, the amazing ability of man and animals to adapt to their surroundings, and the seeming endlessness of the Universe compel many people to seek out answers they feel provide them with some understanding of the nature of things.

I have come to believe that it's not so important *what* you believe, as that you believe *something*. I know there are many people who will not subscribe to this opinion, and that's OK. Again, if you are on a spiritual path that provides you with hope and comfort, that's wonderful. Stay the course—do what feeds your spirit. But—if you're not there yet, I believe the path is actually more important than the destination. It's more important that you are searching, and that you are living a life that allows you to look in the mirror and like the person you see. Keep searching—keep exploring the many belief systems—and don't be afraid to find your own unique path.

The important thing is that it provides you with peace of mind, some clue to the riddle of the meaning of life, and the conviction that you are living a good and honest life.

Support Groups

"I have heard there are troubles of more than one kind.
Some come from ahead and some come from behind.
But I've bought a big bat. I'm all ready you see.
Now my troubles are going to have troubles with me!"
~Dr. Seuss

There are two ways to approach a support group—find one, or start one. If there is a Fibromyalgia support group in your area, I highly recommend checking it out. If there is not a support group in your area, you might want to consider starting one.

Support groups can provide invaluable benefits to people with Fibromyalgia, as they will put you in touch with people to whom you never have to explain yourself. They already know a lot of what you're living with, and they will understand the challenges of living with chronic pain.

If you do not have a local support group, and you are considering whether you should start one, there are some questions you must answer. First, is there a need? If you live in a large metropolitan area, I can almost guarantee the answer to that question is "yes." If you're in a smaller town or a sparsely populated rural area, the answer might be a bit more difficult to quantify. The only way to find out may be to start it and see what kind of response and attendance you get. As a place to start, I recommend you check out www.meetup.com, which has tools with which you can start a basic on-line group, including a calendar and automatic notification to members whenever an event/meeting is added. For a start-up group, it offers a great deal of functionality for a reasonable cost—far less than if you started up a website on your own or paid a web developer to design one. If your group takes off and grows, that can come later, if necessary.

You need to consider whether you have the time and the energy to facilitate such a group. There will be planning, publicity, and attending meetings where you will be the point person. You need to be comfortable speaking in front of groups, as well as comfortable approaching others who might speak to the group. You must be comfortable with facilitating the group, which means keeping the discussion on topic, tactfully cutting off members who want to dominate the discussion or be argumentative, and at the same time ensuring that attendees get the support that they have a right to expect. You are the person others will look to as a role model. If your attitude stinks, so will the attitude of the group. If you are negative, the group will be negative.

It is vital to the health and survival of a support group that the atmosphere be one of positive support and problem-solving. If you allow the group to become a 90-minute bitch-fest, members may participate at first, because they have not previously been able to express their feelings to someone who understands. It is freeing and validating to vent in an atmosphere of support and understanding. But—and this is a big but—that atmosphere must not be allowed to take over the meeting, or members will not continue to attend. In the end, we all seek solutions.

Another consideration is whether you have someone who can help you with the work, and who can be there if you can't. Everyone has an emergency or a conflict now and then, whether it is a child who has to be picked up, your own illness that keeps you at home, or any number of other reasons that you cannot be at a meeting. You need someone who can share the work, and lead the group on short notice if you can't be there. It's important that the person who helps out has the same philosophy and outlook in their approach to

Fibromyalgia, and their outlook on life in general. They must be positive, upbeat, nonjudgmental, and a good listener (qualities you must also have).

Once you have those "pieces" in place, you have some additional decisions to make. You need to identify your target group. Will you only support people with Fibromyalgia, or will you invite people with other chronic pain conditions to join? Will you allow friends, family, and caregivers to attend meetings? While welcoming family and/or friends can be helpful to group members, it may also create an atmosphere where members don't feel entirely free to share their feelings—so you need to weigh the benefits against the possible complications.

It's also important to give a name to your group that will identify the target demographic you seek to serve. The name of the group can be very basic, such as <City> Fibromyalgia Support Group, or you can make it catchy, for instance, the Foggy Fibro Support Group (OK that was lame but you get the idea).

How often you will meet, and where, are the next questions to answer. Some public libraries have meeting rooms that are either free of charge, or only charge a minimal fee. Many churches also allow community groups to use their facilities. It's easier to arrange that if you are a church member, but some churches will open their doors to community groups without the involvement of a church member. One thing that is very important is choosing a day and time for the meeting and sticking with it. Once you have people attending regularly, they will plan around it and make themselves available if they're interested in participating. If you are constantly changing the day and time, and trying to find the "perfect" meeting schedule, it's unfair to those who are already attending, and it's confusing for new members. Don't do this one by "committee"—choose a day and time that works for *you*, and others will follow. If you find out early on that you picked a day that's really bad for most other people, then change it, but only if it really isn't working for your members.

The location must be convenient for you. This is one of those times when it's good to be selfish. You will be the one doing the work, setting the schedule, arranging for speakers if you choose to have them, and you have the right to make the location convenient for you. As time goes on, you may find members who are willing to start a support group in a different part of the area. Then, and only then, you may branch out to offer more dates and times for your members, where you do not have to personally attend. Your time, and your energy, are precious. Don't choose locations and set schedules that cause you stress—that's a sure path to burnout and failure.

Last, but certainly not least, you must identify your mission. Is it to educate and inform, to raise awareness in the community, to raise money for research? You have to know your "why," or the group will flounder around like a ship without a rudder.

A note on fund-raising—if you are a small group with volunteer helpers, you may not need to raise money, as you and/or a few others may be willing to share the costs of handouts (and refreshments if you choose to have them), whether you're purchasing them or making them yourself. If you want to go beyond a minimal amount of expense, consider applying to the IRS to become a 501(c)(3) non-profit, to create a vehicle for the money, and to keep it tax free. Keep in mind that there may be tax consequences for you if you are fund-raising without the umbrella of a registered non-profit organization.

Running a support group can be extremely rewarding, but it does require a significant amount of time and work. Before you go there, just be sure you're prepared.

Attitude

"It is a waste of time to be angry about my disability. One has to get on with life and I haven't done badly. People won't have time for you if you are always angry or complaining." ~Stephen Hawking

"Life is short." We hear that said so often, but we don't really give it a lot of thought most of the time. In the end, most of the things we spend the most emotional energy on turn out to be small stuff. When things aren't going your way, before you panic, ask yourself these questions: Will it matter in five minutes? Five days? Five years? The first question is probably the only one you need for most situations, but if the answer to that first question is "yes" then proceed to the next question, and the next, until you satisfy yourself that the situation in question is really important enough to warrant your time and energy.

It doesn't matter how much or how little you have. What matters is how you perceive it. It's sometimes tempting to judge people by what they own, but that's often only a measure of how much they've spent, or worse, how much debt they have. Adjust your perspective from "Wow I wish I had her house…." to "Wow I'm sure glad I don't have her mortgage payment!" or "I'm so grateful my little house is so easy to maintain!" If you can make that adjustment, you'll find yourself much more content with what you have, and less envious of others.

Things aren't important. Love, Kindness, Justice, Friends, and Family are important. No one ever lay on their deathbed smiling about how much "stuff" they accumulated in their lifetime. When you read or hear that a person died "surrounded by friends and family," that's important.

Don't sweat the small stuff—and most of what you encounter in life is ultimately small stuff. In the words of Sheryl Crow, "…it's not having what you want, it's wanting what you've got."

Counseling

You cannot teach a man anything. You can only help him discover it within himself. ~Galileo Galilei

This can be a sore subject for people with Fibromyalgia. So many misunderstandings, miscommunications, and myths surround the whole issue of Fibromyalgia that it's often difficult to know what's real. One thing that contributes to the misunderstandings is that anti-depressants are a common medication choice for Fibromyalgia. This leads a lot of Fibromyalgia patients to think that their doctor believes the pain is "all in their head." The other easy assumption is that your doctor thinks you're "just depressed." Neither of these is typically the case, but it's easy to see how the misunderstandings start.

Doctors—most doctors anyway—are not taught good communication skills. They learn how to treat the body, but not how to treat the whole person. The doctor says "take this and you'll feel better," and we hear "you're just depressed—take this antidepressant and you'll feel better." What they should be saying is more like "this medication is often prescribed as an antidepressant, but it works by increasing the amount of available serotonin and norepinephrine, two neurotransmitter chemicals in your brain that are thought to have an effect on pain 'messages' and how the brain processes them. By that chemical action, this drug may help with your Fibromyalgia pain."

Another issue of misunderstanding surrounds the recommendation and use of Cognitive Behavioral Therapy for people with Fibromyalgia. When a doctor recommends that a Fibromyalgia patient see a counselor, again, the patient may hear "you're just depressed—talk to someone and you'll feel better." That is generally not what your doctor meant—the reason Cognitive Behavioral Therapy is recommended in Fibromyalgia has much more to do with the many life adjustments, both mental and physical, that must be made by someone who has been told that they have an incurable condition. While Fibromyalgia is not life-threatening, it is often life-altering. Cognitive Behavioral Therapy can help with the adjustments that must be made, and can smooth the path in ways that will differ for each person, depending on what obstacles they encounter in their journey with Fibromyalgia.

This is another of those times when I have to say I don't know you, but I do know that there are very few people who would not benefit from talking with a compassionate counselor from time to time. In the interest of full disclosure, I will tell you that I practice what I preach. I have been in counseling several times in my life, and whatever success I have had in building a good life, I attribute in great part to the assistance of the three remarkable women who have, at different times, been my counselor.

Resources

Some good websites for Fibromyalgia information:

National Fibromyalgia Association
www.fmaware.org

Fibromyalgia Network
www.fmnetnews.com

American Chronic Pain Association
http://www.theacpa.org/

Fibromyalgia Support
http://www.fibromyalgia-support.org

Mayo Clinic
http://www.mayoclinic.com

DailyStrength—A Support Website
http://www.dailystrength.org

The Dragon Grins

By Ray White, 1997

The doctor explains to me that I have a Dragon that has come to possess me. This Dragon is mean. This Dragon is deceiving and destructive. "But", the doctor says, "We can work at keeping this Dragon down."

"What is this Dragon's name?" I ask.

The doctor in his professional calmness says, "The Dragon is FMS…Fibromyalgia Syndrome" The doctor explains to me ways we are going to keep him down. "Feed the Dragon some meds like Trazadone or Elavil. Do some light exercise, maybe the Dragon will get tired and leave you alone for a while."

I turn to leave and for the first time I see the Dragon. He looks at me with those evil yellow eyes, and the Dragon grins. I say to myself that Dragons can be slain. I read that in stories in school. The armor-clad knight slaying the Dragon and triumphantly returning to his town. As I am in this daydream the Dragon jumps on me. I wrestle with him. His hot breath sears my head. His roar makes my ears ring. He leaves me in a pile of flesh on the ground. I ache all over. Some parts of my body are painful to touch. I am exhausted as I pick myself back up again. The Dragon looks back to me-and the Dragon grins.

"I hate you, Dragon." I scream as he walks away. I feed the Dragon the medication prescribed. Slowly at first, then increasing a little as time goes by. I do begin a little exercise. I change some of my diet and increase the carbohydrates. I move about relatively pain free. And I say to myself "Maybe I have beaten the Dragon. Maybe the Dragon was only my imagination. I was just a little depressed and down, but now life is great."

I look to the sky and see dark clouds looming. A cold north wind begins to blow. I hear a thunderous pounding of foot steps. I have heard that sound while watching Jurassic Park, but now I'm not watching that movie. BOOM…BOOM…I don't see anything. BOOM…BOOM. I panic and start to run. I don't know where to run, but I run. The pounding gets closer and louder. I feel the hot breath on my neck. I dare not turn around as I try to run faster…faster. A claw grabs my shoulder. Searing hot pain rips down my back….staring upwards, terror runs through my body. And the Dragon grins.

The Dragon has returned! "You can't escape" the Dragon yells, "You are mine !!" I try to get up as the Dragon slams my body back to the ground. I can hardly stand the pain as he tortures me by stomping my hands. With his teeth he pulls at muscles in my back and legs. He burns my head with intense fiery breath. The battle is finally over. He stares at my crumpled body as I try to get focused on this beast. My eyes finally clear enough to see, and the Dragon grins.

Days pass. My fingers no longer work like they used to. My muscles feel like the second day of Olympic training, but the sensation does not leave. My head is not clear. I do not see well at night. Parts of me are cold and clammy. I am stiff. Why did the Dragon beat me so hard? When I try to sleep, the Dragon slaps me awake several times at night. Sometimes I am freezing. In bed I awaken drenched in sweat. It hurts to stand. It hurts to sit. My mind says one thing and my mouth says another. And the Dragon grins.

Sometimes I think I am in a nightmare and will someday wake up, the real me. I don't look sick, so why do I feel so bad? Friends and family laugh when I mess up on my words talking to them. I feel stupid looking in the refrigerator and not knowing why, or walking around in circles either not finding what I was after or forgetting what I was looking for. If I am driving at night and it starts to rain, the road disappears. And it is not uncommon to go somewhere and then make wrong turns coming back. My mind says right, my body turns left. I can go somewhere and not remember how I got there. I am not dumb, just not "connected" anymore.

Outwardly I laugh and play, but inside I have to cry sometimes.

And the Dragon grins.

Lightning Source UK Ltd.
Milton Keynes UK
UKOW050629130512

192468UK00001B/19/P